I0479141

Dietary Deficiencies in Tinnitus and Hearing Impairment

By

Lynne D M Noble

Independently published 2023

About the Author

Lynne Noble was born in 1953 in Huddersfield, West Yorkshire. From a very early age, Lynne showed an interest in nutrition and genetics avidly reading any books that she could get her hands on at the time.

Initially, Lynne studied orthopaedics but events led her to work with the elderly mentally infirm. Here, her interest in neurodegenerative disorders and pain syndromes developed.

Lynne undertook rigorous programmes of study, completing her Cert Ed., (FE) BSc (Hons) and Adv. Dip Education simultaneously before moving onto her M.Ed.

From there she took further demanding programmes in Human Nutrition, Pharmacology, Neuroscience, Genetics and Immunology. During this time, she was given many prestigious awards for her academic work. It was noted then that Lynne was not afraid of tackling difficult subjects.

She began her law degree but ill health prevented her from pursuing this. However, in this time, she moved from being a foster parent to adoptive parent.

She has been instrumental in setting up projects in the community for disadvantaged groups.

She is a member of the Guild of Health Writers.

Now retired, she lives with her husband in a historic Georgian riverside town in the West Midlands. She enjoys gardening, watching her husband bowling and researching.

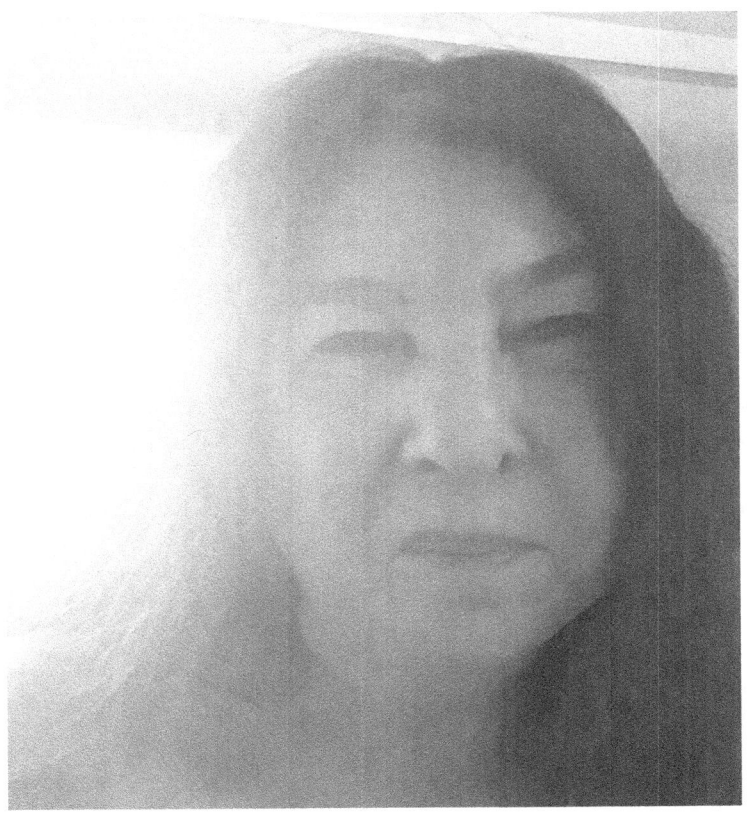

Author Lynne Noble at home

Table of Contents

Tinnitus

You hiss and shriek, constant, unending

Bending my thoughts to this cacophony

Instead of the way of glorious silence.

A demented Vespa, without conscience

Curses its profanity inside my head

Seething, uncaring, there is no rest

From this ungodly uninvited guest

L D M Noble 2023

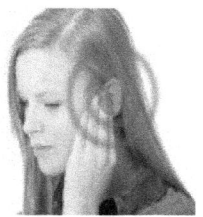

Preface

One of the things that I have learned with my interactions with others on social media is how distressing tinnitus is. The second piece of information I have learned is that it is not taken seriously by the medical profession, or others, yet its impact can have serious consequences including depression, insomnia and social isolation.

Finally, I learned that there appears to be little help for those who do suffer from this distressing condition both in terms of what caused it and how it can be alleviated.

Although the subject of my next book was intended to be an entirely different subject, I turned my attention to the subject of tinnitus, being drawn to it because of the huge numbers of sufferers who did not appear to have anywhere to turn.

I am thankful that I do not have any chronic condition that I have been informed I must 'put up with for the rest of my life' or it is part of the ageing process and therefore there is nothing that can be done. How sad and dispiriting these statements are especially as they are also untrue.

Most readers will know my views on the current thinking of the ageing process. The ageing process does not result in chronic disease and illness. Chronic disease and illness occur because the equilibrium in the human body has been disturbed, for whatever reason, and once the underlying cause has been established then it can be corrected with partial or whole recovery.

Throughout the book I will give the voices of those suffering from tinnitus a voice which will be emboldened and italicised.

As always, my main focus is on treating conditions with good nutrition although therapeutic treatment with supplements may be advised for a short period.

What is Tinnitus?

A friend of my daughter went to his doctor seeking help for the tinnitus he's had for a couple of years. Best his doctor could offer him was to sever his auditory nerve rendering him basically deaf

Tinnitus is generally described as a sound that is not coming from an external source and can include ringing, clicking, buzzing, hissing, roaring like an ocean. It can be thunderous or soft, high pitched whining or low pitched groaning. People experience it in many ways but no one agrees that it is easy to live with.

Tinnitus may appear in just one ear but later it may occur in the other ear too. Sometimes it appears to go away and then returns with a vengeance.

I've had tinnitus since 2004, was mild at first. Now its constant, just my left side. It's so loud and high pitched. It affects my hearing and concentration. Sometimes I get like a banging sound, like 3 big bags in among it. I gave up going to docs, was told to put white noise on.

John

So, now we have established that tinnitus is a wide range of noises that do not have an external source. The noises occur because of something that has gone wrong with some internal functioning. However, the cause is not a singular one. There appear to be many causes with each having their own particular route to be taken to reverse the condition. Some will be easier to address than others so the initial part of the process in understanding your particular tinnitus is to investigate the reasons underpinning it.

However, in order to understand tinnitus better, it would be judicious to investigate if there are any groups which it appears to affect more than others.

I've had tinnitus for around 15 years in my left ear. I try not to focus on it, but some days it's hard! You have my sympathy.

Geordie at heart

Research[1] has shown that tinnitus occurs in about 15% of people aged between 40-80 years world-wide with a peak of chronic tinnitus peaking for those aged between 60-69 yrs.

This should not really surprise us given that hearing loss tends to be more common as age

---

[1] https://www.ncbi.nlm.nih.gov/pmc/articles/PMC5187663/

increases and hearing loss is also a well-established risk factor for tinnitus.

However, it should be born in mind that not all those suffering from hearing loss will go on to suffer from tinnitus so clearly a risk factor is not causation and further investigation is often required.

Tinnitus is not classed as a disease. It is considered to be a symptom that something, somewhere is wrong in the auditory system.

The auditory system consists of the outer ear known as the pinna, and the auditory nerve which connects the inner ear to the brain. The brain of course processes sound in many areas of the brain.

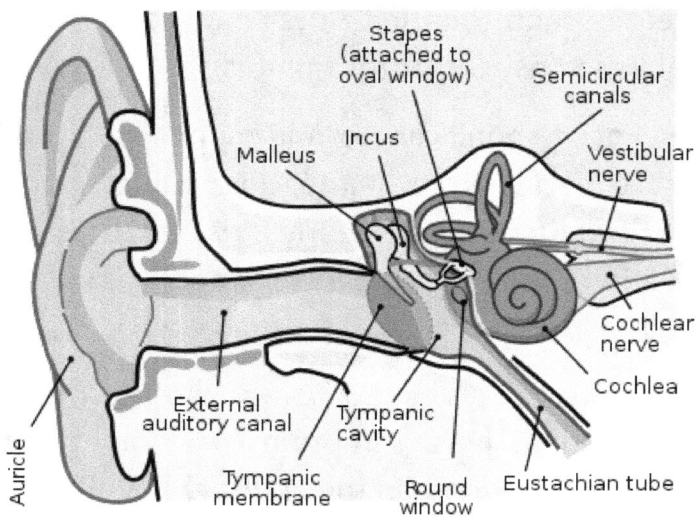

The auditory system

The temporal lobe of the brain is where nerve signals travel to and are interpreted as sound.

The signals cross over so that sounds from the right ear travel to the cortex dealing with sound on the left temporal lobe and vice versa.

The job of these cortices is much that of a personal assistant. They file, process, interpret and file all the information received about the sound.

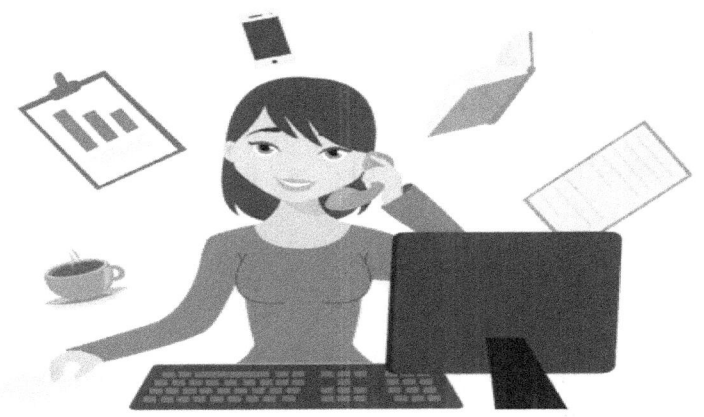

The auditory cortex files, processes, interprets and files all information held about the incoming sound. In this respect it is not much different from the job a personal assistant has.

As tinnitus is only a symptom then the causes can range from something as simple as ear wax blockage – which is relatively easy to address, once you are aware of it- to other more complex causes.

These will be explored along with any causative nutritional deficiencies - or excess - and are listed below.

Thyroid abnormalities

Brain tumours

Ear wax blockage

Noise induced hearing loss

Ear and sinus infections

Meniere's disease

Diseases of the heart or blood vessels

Medications – of which more than 200 medications contribute

Hearing loss

Now that this has been established, I shall take them in order to see what can be done about the reasons underpinning tinnitus.

Thyroid abnormalities

The thyroid is a small gland which sits just in front of the windpipe, also known as the trachea. It is butterfly shaped.

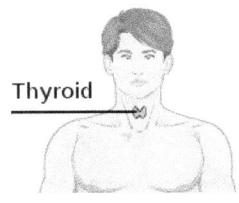

Thyroid

It produces hormone. Hormones are chemical messengers which travel to the site where they are needed. Thyroid hormones affect things like body temperature and heart rate. An excess or deficiency can cause some very unpleasant symptoms indeed.

Hypothyroidism is the less common manifestation of thyroid dysfunction. Often underdiagnosed in those whose symptoms are vague, this condition tends to occur in women more than men.

The clinical symptoms of hypothyroidism include cognitive changes, which may include inability to focus and multitask, or forgetfulness. Cold intolerance, weight gain, constipation and the appearance of a goitre – which is the enlargement of the thyroid gland - may be seen.

Prevalence increases with age which is consistent with the greater likelihood of hearing loss with the associated risk of tinnitus.

Hashimoto's is the most common cause of hypothyroidism which is an inflammatory condition. The tinnitus attached to Hashimoto's is generally heard as a continuous sound.

Noticeable tinnitus started with my Hashimoto's thyroiditis. Worked out it's a top C! Can't spend much time in a silent atmosphere like an abbey or cathedral as it builds and feels like an internal pressure. Very sad I'll never experience complete silence again.

Sophie A

Patients with autoimmune Hashimoto's are at risk of developing other autoimmune conditions. In this case an autoimmune inner ear disease (AIED) develops which attacks the inner ear. Any inflammation of the nerve here can lead to symptoms of tinnitus.

While most people hear Hashimoto's tinnitus as a continuous whine, it may initially fluctuate before progressing. In some cases, there may be sudden hearing loss in one or both ears.

In my book, The Thyroid Diet[2], I explore how diet may address Hashimoto's thyroiditis through understanding the role of excessive iodine, goitregens and other substances which impact the smooth operation of the thyroid gland.

These are rarely, if ever, discussed or recommended in the doctor's surgery. Auto immunity may respond very well to changes in the diet with vitamin D which is known as the immunomodulatory vitamin. It helps regulate the immune system so that it does not go into overdrive or does not function sub-optimally, either.

---

[2] https://www.amazon.co.uk/dp/B0BXNPBTQR

Approximately 80% of the world population are deficient in this vitamin which is required for strong bones as well as regulating inflammation.

It is one of the most difficult of vitamins to take in sufficient quantities through the diet. Foods containing vitamin D are limited and what foods there are do not contain great amounts. As we get older we are less likely to absorb the nutrients from our diet. Vitamin D is no different so increasing age is a risk factor for a deficiency of vitamin D.

Most of our vitamin D is taken in through the action of the sun's rays on the skin but even this process becomes less efficient as we age.

Supplementation of 4000 IU's is recommended daily but vitamin D requires it to be taken with a little fat for bioavailability. In addition, magnesium is required for activation of vitamin D.

Also bear in mind that the form of vitamin D should be the active form D3 rather than the inactive form, D2. The requires a number of steps to be converted to the active form. As age progresses, the conversion process is likely to be less effective resulting in a deficiency.

Dietary sources of vitamin D are irradiated mushrooms, eggs and oily fish.

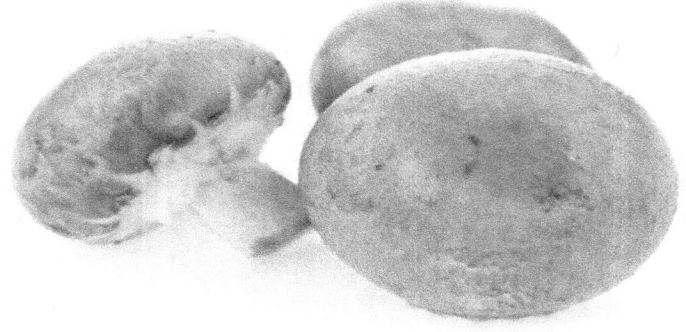

Mushrooms, when left in the sun, make a small amount of vitamin D. It is the inactive form of vitamin D2.

Cholesterol is required for the synthesis of vitamin D from the sun's rays, so statin users are at a disadvantage when their cholesterol levels are artificially lowered.

Vitamin D receptors are found in every organ system of the body thus showing its impact on whole body health.   The best food sources of vitamin D are found in the table below.   Lest anyone think that they can tweak their diet to take in sufficient vitamin D when taking statins, I would say that this is highly unlikely.

Cholesterol is also needed to make bile without which the fat soluble vitamins cannot absorbed. A possible condition that may manifest itself that most people would not think would be linked to tinnitus or hearing impairment, is gall bladder inflammation and stones. However, bile is needed to break down and emulsify fats and vitamin D is needed to make bile. How exquisitely our body systems interact.

Three hours of sunlight (in the UK) between the beginning of May and the end of September will produce about the minimum requirement of vitamin Daily. Clearly, this will increase if fewer items of clothing are worn.

In winter light, exposure with normal clothing results in the synthesis of only 10% of that benefitted from in the summer.

Table showing the best food sources of vitamin D

Best food sources showing micrograms per 100g of food

Cod liver oil	**210**
kippers	**210**
mackerel	**17.50**
Canned salmon	**12.50**
Sardines	**7.50**
Tuna fresh not tinned	**5.80**
eggs	**1.75**
milk	**0.03**

Lard is, of course, a superfood and contains 102 micrograms of vitamin D in 100g of lard. Of course, we do not eat great amounts of lard – even less so when the allegedly healthier oils have elbowed them out of place – and this is a great shame as lard has enormous benefits for health.

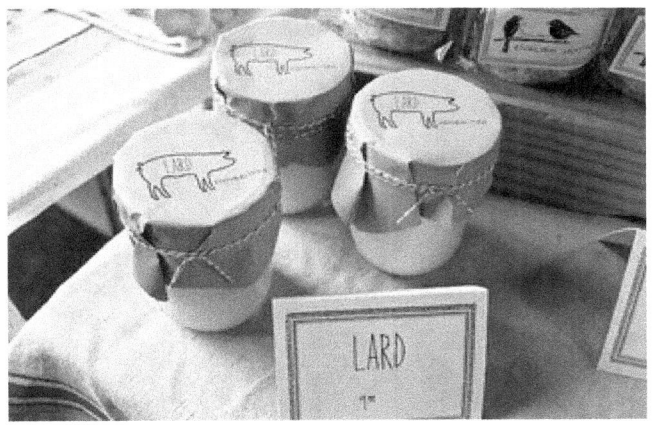

Lard, a much maligned superfood which contains superior amounts of vitamin D. Popular in the 1940's and 1950's it has sadly fallen out of fashion.

Some deficiency symptoms which you need to be aware on in addition to tinnitus are: bone pain, muscular weakness and spasms, and bones which fracture easily.

Vitamin D is a stable vitamin and not easily lost in sunlight, storage or cooking.

The role of taurine in nerve inflammation

Taurine is not an essential amino acid (EAA). It is manufactured in the body although synthesis may be superior in the younger rather than the older individual. It is not found in vegetable protein.

It is synthesised from two sulphur containing amino acids – methionine and cysteine. It is synthesised in the liver but needs vitamin B6 to be present to assist this process.

The female estradiol inhibits the formation of taurine in the liver.

Taurine in sufficient doses is found to stimulate the production of growth hormone. Human growth hormone is called an anabolic hormone. An anabolic hormone helps to build up tissue as opposed to catabolic hormones which break tissue down. Therefore, HGH builds as well as repairs tissues.

Can taurine repair damaged nerves which may be contributing to the symptoms of tinnitus in thyroid disease? Well, there is plenty of research to support this too.

So, what is the dosage of taurine that may resolve many of the damages caused to nerves?

The dosage is:
1g for the first day

500mg for the next seven days
50mg-100mg thereafter.

High alcohol consumption and the use of salicylates like aspirin can decrease taurine. Other disorders may also decrease taurine. These include: myocardial infarction, fractures or other bone disorders, stress, blood disorders and a deficiency of zinc.

Taurine has been found to reverse the suppression of thyroid function.

The best sources of taurine – which can only be found in animal protein – is oily fish.

Noisy environments

Noisy environments are well known for causing hearing impairment. Those particularly at risk are individuals who work in noisy environments which include musicians and construction workers.

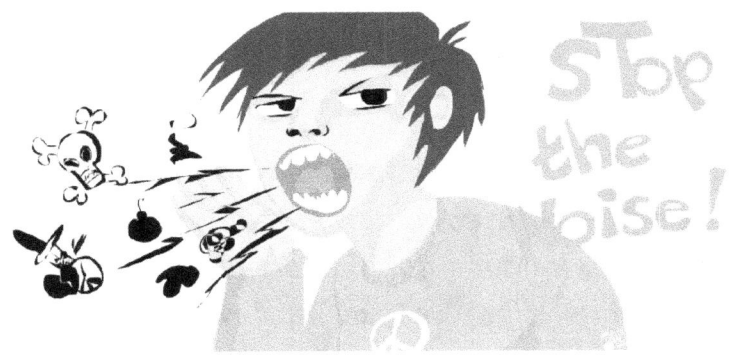

Any exposure to noise will damage the tiny sensory hairs in the inner ear. These tiny hairs help transmit sound to the brain where it is interpreted into speech or other sounds.

We refer to this damage as noise-induced hearing loss and it was particularly common in the 1960's when rock bands became popular but ear defenders had not yet been invented.

Constant whooshing in my both ears and constant itch. It's as if I can hear my blood flow. If I hold a specific bit on my neck the sound goes away obv can't hold it for long lol.

Every time I mention it to the doctor he says ok and gives me an ear drop which does nothing.

Caz

This is me it seems, mine is constant high pitch ringing in both ears, sometimes one will pop and go louder it is horrible and very distracting. If you've ever had ringing in your ears after a night out it's similar to that.

Deb

Mine started after I worked in construction.

Tom

There   is a rare type of tinnitus which sounds like pulsing and it appears to harmonise with your heartbeat.   It is called pulsatile tinnitus. There are a number of reasons why this may be so.

Firstly, abnormalities in the structure of the brain may cause this rhythmic pulsing. Brain tumours, in some cases, are responsible for this rhythmic quality.

With some manifestations of tinnitus, it is fairly easy to understand why the symptoms of tinnitus may have occurred. People can understand that damage has occurred due to the exposure of excessive and prolonged noise or structural abnormalities or the formation of a tumour.

Exposure to noise often results in the loss of sensory hair cells. The neural circuits adapt to this loss by increasing sensitivity to sound. The downshoot of this is that some individuals with tinnitus can become overly sensitive to sound.

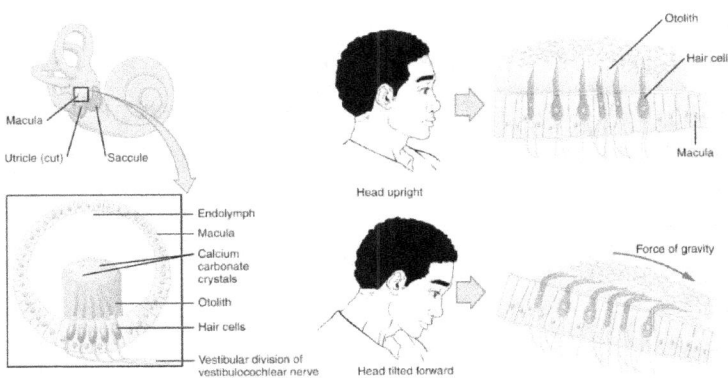

The noise that we think is in our ears is actually interpreted in our neural circuits. This is similar to the pain we feel in our hands or lower limbs.

The damage may occur in those areas but the pain is actually felt in the neural circuits. The neural circuits actually make sense of the sound waves that originate externally to us.

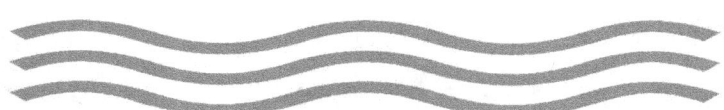

Sound waves are not interpreted until they reach the auditory cortex in the brain. Prior to that they are just vibrations travelling along the auditory nerve.

One of the theories is that when damage has occurred at some point, the brain remembers the 'pain' of the damage (rather like phantom limb pain) and continues to replay the sound distortions long after the original injury has healed. We know that if we have had an ear infection that sound may be distorted or we feel pressure not unlike we do when taking off in an aeroplane. While most people recall the feeling on one level as a memory, it is not generally accompanied by the physical feeling of discomfort. However, some people do have a continuous sound in their ears just as some people with amputated limbs can feel pain in the lost limb and others can't.

Neural circuits do interact with each other and sometimes they do not do it as well as they used to. We do not hear of children complaining of tinnitus. It seems very much to be a symptom which sojourns with adults.

Maybe when damage occurs, due to excessive exposure to sound, the injury inflicted throws all signalling activity out of synchronisation in the auditory cortex where sound is eventually processed into something we intelligible to us. Sound is merely waves or nervous impulses. It is the auditory cortex which interprets these waves.

So, in a nutshell, from the external ear to the brain there are a lot of things that can go wrong but most likely prolonged exposure to sound will damage the tiny hairs which then, like a roll of dominoes, have a knock on effect on the rest of the system or have 'learned' the sounds from the original damage caused and are regurgitating it whether you like it or not.

The sensory receptor cells in the cochlea may be more sensitive to damage in some individuals because they are low in vitamin A. The cochlea needs a high concentration of vitamin A in order for these special cells to be able to function[3]

It appears that low serum vitamin A is a risk factor for decreased auditory function.

Phantom Pain occurs when there is pain in the part of the body which has been removed. Some patients may feel pain in their leg even after it has been amputated.

This occurs because whenever an injury occurs, pain is registered in the brain and creates a physical neurological pathway. Even after a limb is amputated the pathway is still there with its potential for feeling pain.

On a smaller scale, all pain as a result of injury will create a neurological pathway where it is registered.

---

[3] *Chole Q. Vitamin A in the cochlea. Arch. Otorhinolaryngol. 124:379-82, 1978*

This will become more entrenched the longer an injury remains unhealed. It is therefore of great importance that pain is addressed as soon as is possible. The stoic among us, who do not resort attempt to alleviate pain, may be troubled with long standing pain as a result of the neurological pathways which have 'captured' the pain resulting from the injury.

What are the sources of vitamin A? It is found only in foods of animal origin such as cod liver oils, cheese and eggs. However, there is a precursor in beta-carotene known as beta-carotene and we are familiar with beta-carotene in orange fruit and vegetables such as carrots and pumpkin.

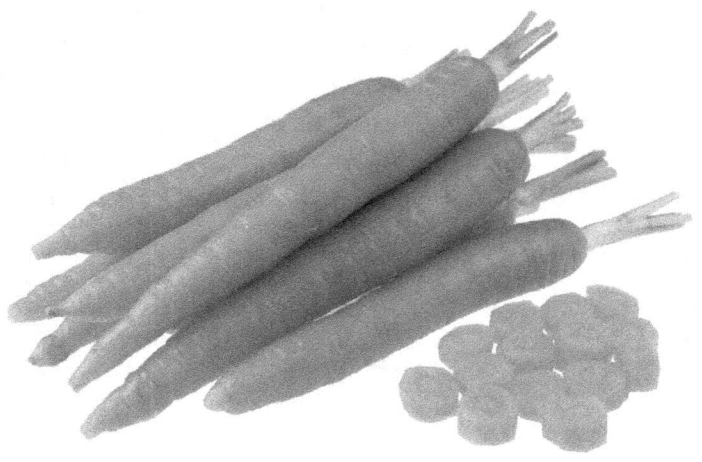

Carrots contain beta carotene, the precursor to vitamin A. Beta carotene needs to be taken with a little fat for it to be absorbed, hence the practice of adding a little butter before serving.

The absorption of beta-carotene is enhanced by a little fat in the diet. In these days of low fat and no fat diets, it is clear that a vitamin A deficiency is quite probable.

Food fortification of vitamin A occurs when retinyl palmitate and retinyl acetate are added.

Best food source of fat soluble vitamin A (micrograms per 100g)

Food type	Micrograms/100g
Halibut liver oil	60,000
Liver	18,000
butter	750
Cheese	385
eggs	140

750 mcg or 25000 IU's of vitamin A is the recommended daily intake.

As vitamin A is required for optimum health of the auditory and visual organs, mucous membranes, acts as an anti-infective, anti-anaemia agent and is required for protein synthesis and growth, it is not surprising that some of the deficiency symptoms include:

Eye ulceration

Dry eyes

Eyeball pain

Burning and itching eyes

Poor sight

Spinal infections

Respiratory infection

Scaly skin and scalp

Poor hair quality

Night blindness

Kidney stones

Inflamed mucous membranes

Tinnitus

As vitamin A is a fat soluble vitamin, supplementation is not recommended as excess intake is a possibility. Nevertheless, supplementary daily intake, if necessary for therapeutic reasons for short periods only, should not exceed 2250 mcg or 7500 IU's.

However, vitamin A deficiency is not the only nutrient that may damage the tiny cochlear hair cells. A deficiency of magnesium is also a risk factor for such.

Magnesium deficiency has a role in hearing impairment and tinnitus

In a 1983 study[4] it was put forward that aminoglycoside drugs caused ototoxicity by depleting magnesium in the hair cells.

---

[4] *Dolov E et al. Is magnesium depletion the reason for ototoxicity caused by aminoglycosides? Med Hypotheses 10 (4): 353-58, 1983*

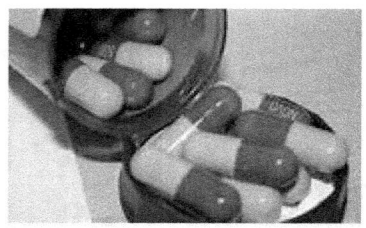

Aminoglycoside drugs cause ototoxicity by depleting magnesium in hair cells

Magnesium deficiency is rife in society. The body contains approximately 25g of magnesium which is distributed widely in bones, organs nerves and blood.

It is difficult to measure magnesium levels as there is little in serum. Most is contained in cells and cost inhibits routine tests for it.

Magnesium is a cofactor in many bodily process including the production of energy, cell replication. It is a cofactor in hormones, stabilises cell structure, a component of chlorophyll, is require for nerve impulse transmission and a cofactor for two very important B vitamins thiamine (B1) and pyroxidone (B6). This is just the tip of the iceberg really.

You can understand that if magnesium is required for nerve impulses that a magnesium deficiency could well result in tinnitus.

Indeed, there are many reasons that could cause a magnesium deficiency which include:

Poor dietary intake

Malnutrition

Anorexia

High dietary intake of vitamin D, vitamin B1, calcium and saturated fats.

Reduced absorption due to antacids (especially PPI's) laxative abuse, diuretics, allergies, infections, kidney disease, alcoholism, diabetes, cancer, antibiotics, drugs for the cardiovascular system, the contraceptive pill and a high milk intake diet.

The results of the above may result in deficiency symptoms alongside tinnitus such as:

Painful swallowing

Low blood sugar

Palpitations

Arrhythmia

Hyperactivity

Unsteadiness on feet

Nystagmus

Weakness, tiredness, general lassitude

Dizziness

Anxiety

Convulsions

Muscle cramps and tremors

And many more….

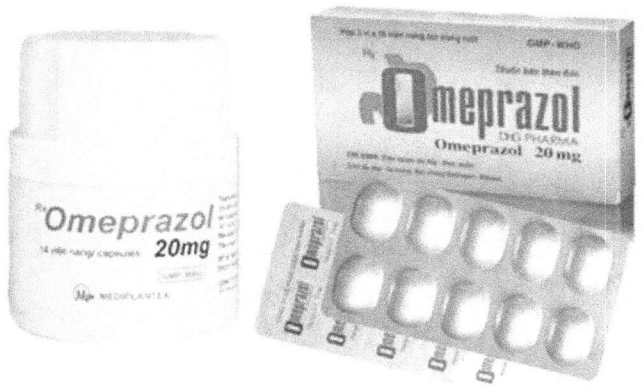

Omeprazole may inhibit magnesium absorption and, as such be indirectly a risk factor for hearing impairment and tinnitus.

Fortunately, magnesium is found in many foods. These can be found in the table below.

Best sources of magnesium in mg/100g

Soya beans	310mg
nuts	250mg
Dried brewer's yeast	230mg
Dried peas	117mg
seafoods	90mg
meats	50mg

bananas	42mg
Green leafy vegetables	25mg

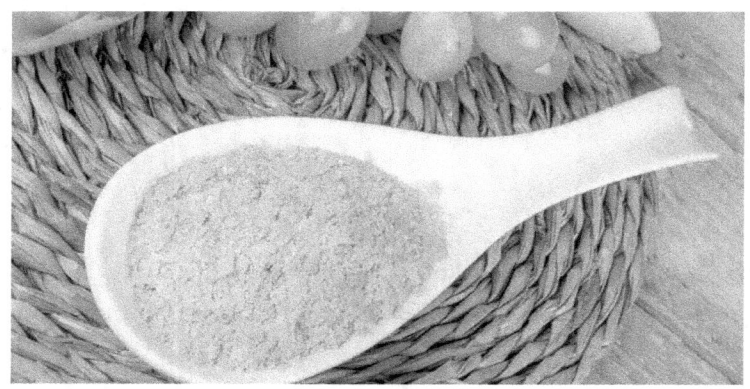

Dried brewer's yeast is an excellent source of magnesium.

The recommended daily intake of magnesium is 400mg but, of course, this would depend on other factors such as whether diuretics are being taken or magnesium absorption is inhibited by the use of PPI's, for example.

The neural circuits do not exist in isolation from other regions in the brain either. They, for example, are intimately connected with the limbic system.

The limbic system regulates mood and emotion so it is not surprising that people under severe or prolonged stress may also report tinnitus as one of their symptoms.

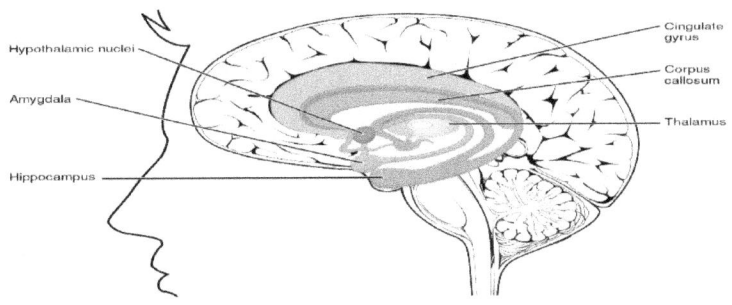

The limbic system has an association with tinnitus as well as mood and emotion

Stress, high blood sugar levels and tinnitus

Stressful events can, and do, result in tinnitus. Stress causes adrenalin release which results in vasoconstriction in the inner ear.   Reactive hypoglycaemia often occurs with a high carbohydrate meal and consequent adrenaline release. In this case, the tinnitus is often accompanied by hearing loss.

The hearing loss will be fluctuating as you would expect with reactive blood sugar levels.

An observational study [5]of 90 patients found that 58% of those with sensorineural hearing loss had abnormal 5 hour glucose tolerance tests.

Another observational study found that 42% of 19 patients with Meniere's syndrome showed hypoglycaemia at some point in a 5 hr glucose tolerance test compared to 15% of patents with other disease (Weille FR *Hypoglycaemia in Meniere's disease. Arch. Oto I*87:129.1968).

Apart from tinnitus, other studies have shown that headache and vertigo are associated with a hypoglycaemic tendency.

Diabetics may be prone to this type of tinnitus and hearing loss. Of course, our ability to deal with high carbohydrate meals becomes less

---

[5] Yanick P Grosselin EJ. Audiologic and metabolic findings in 90 patients with fluctuant hearing loss. !. Am Audiol, Soc 2:15-18, 1975

effective as we age and may well correlate with the increase in tinnitus and hearing loss as we age.

Indeed, the incidence of diabetes and heart disease decreases with increasing chromium levels. However, chromium levels do decrease with age.

Keto diets may well ameliorate – or remove – the symptoms of tinnitus but chromium is **the** Glucose Tolerance Factor which those with this underlying cause of tinnitus may well be deficient in.

Not many people understand the role that chromium has to play in balancing blood sugar levels so   it would be wise to add some information about chromium below.

Chromium functions as the glucose tolerance factor – GTF – and no other function has been found for it.

GTF stimulates insulin activity through two actions:

1) It binds to insulin
2) It binds to insulin receptors

Therefore, GTF is able to:

Suppress hunger through the satiety centre

Controls glucose by promoting uptake by muscles and organs

Increases resistance to infection

Stimulated production of essential nerve substances

Stimulated burning of glucose for energy

Stimulates protein synthesis

Controls blood cholesterol levels

Reduces arteriosclerosis (in rat experiments at least)

Reduces fat levels in the blood

In spite of lack of awareness of the role that chromium and GTF play, it has an important role to play in prevent reactive hypoglycaemia and its potential for fluctuant hearing loss.

Absorption of chromium from food is poor. No more than 10% is absorbed, However, when chromium is yeast bound then the absorption rate can increase to 25%. Nevertheless, chromium is excreted in faeces and urine so laxative and diuretic use are detrimental to overall body content.

In order to increase chromium levels without supplementing then including more yeast based products will certainly help. Yeast contains chromium as a GTF and it is 50 times more effective than other types of chromium. It is an even more effective than the chromium found in our superfood, liver.

Brewer's yeast is therefore the 'go to' food if you are diabetic or have reactive hypoglycaemia. We had yeast flakes to our daily diet and love the nutty, savoury taste that enhances our food. However, there are other good food sources and these are found in the table below:

Best food sources of chromium in mcg per 100g (recommended daily intake is 50-200mcg)

Egg yolk	183
molasses	121
Dried brewer's yeast	117
beef	58
Hard cheese	55
liver	55
bran	36
Wheat germ	

There are small amounts of chromium in alcoholic beverages, vegetables and fruit

Deficiency can easily occur with – but are not limited to -

some medicines like diuretics and laxatives

Diets high in carbohydrates and refined foods will create a deficiency.

Prolonged slimming diets

Alcoholism

pregnancy

Symptoms of chromium deficiency

If some of these accompany tinnitus, then it is supports your investigation that blood sugar disturbance is the cause of your tinnitus. The symptoms are very similar to those of hypoglycaemia and include:

Irritability, frustration, an intolerable attitude, mental confusion, depression, lassitude, learning disabilities, anxiety, urinary frequency, thirst, hunger, weight loss and itching.

No symptoms of excess have been recorded.

This concludes our look at chromium and the GTF factor which may have great importance for treating tinnitus and fluctuant hearing loss.

Of course, stress is not just about reactive hypoglycaemia. External events and internal disequilibrium occur for many reasons. External stressors are better dealt with by learning new coping mechanisms. Internal disquiet is often a result of poor nutritional status and although you may not always be able to pinpoint the exact problem, increasing animal fats and protein and reducing carbohydrates in a varied diet will often cure the problem.

Vegetable oils – olive oils excepted – are highly inflammatory in nature and will not help many conditions. They should be steered clear of if at all possible.

Tinnitus may also be found in a condition known as otosclerosis which also has a nutrient deficiency as a probable cause so it is this we will turn to next.

Otosclerosis and vitamin D deficiency as a cause of tinnitus

In a study[6] of 47 patients with otosclerosis, 10 were found to have abnormally low 25-OH vitamin D levels and borderline levels in 2 patients.

Otosclerosis is the abnormal hardening of the ear tissue which is caused by poor remodelling of bone in the middle ear. Bone remodelling occurs as a life-long process but our particular focus is the area that is associated with tinnitus.

A group particularly affected by this underlying cause for tinnitus is white, middle-aged women.

Incoming sound waves vibrate the ear drum. These vibrations travel to three tiny bones in the middle ear known as the

Malleus

Incus

Stapes

which are the Latin names for hammer, anvil and stirrup.

_____

6 *Otolaryngol, Head, Neck, Surg* 93 (3): 313-21, 1985

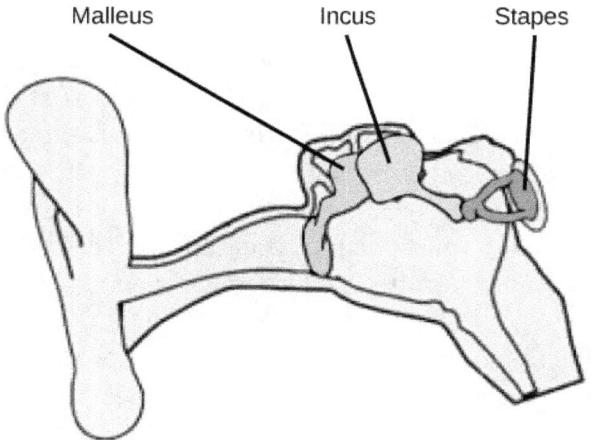

Malleus   Incus   Stapes

Cranial Bones

These bones act as magnifiers, magnifying the vibrations before sending them to the fluid filled cochlea. The upper and lower parts of the cochlear are separated by the basilar, an elastic membrane.

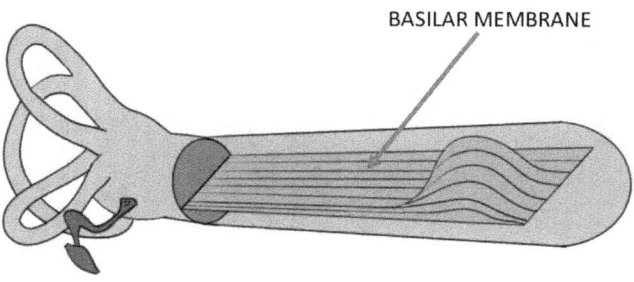

BASILAR MEMBRANE

The vibrations cause the fluid inside to move and the waves travel along the basilar membrane. The hair cells which sit on top of the membrane surf these waves in tandem.

The bristle like hairs then contact the upper membrane and as they tip to one side in the wave, pore like channels open to allow chemicals to rush in. An electrical signal is generated which is then carried by the auditory nerve to the brain.

The end product of this process is recognisable sound.

Otosclerosis – and the accompanying tinnitus – was found to respond significantly to calcium and vitamin D replacement.

The vitamin D supplementation was in the region of 500-1000mg so quite a small dose by today's supplementing recommendations.

Vitamin D is, of course, quite difficult to obtain in any reasonable amount from diet alone and even then, consideration has to be taken of the importance of it to be accompanied by fat and magnesium for absorption and activation, respectively.

Sunlight is the main source of vitamin D but in short supply in the UK. Even if we live in an area where there is a great deal of sunshine, our capacity to make vitamin D is less efficient as we age. We need cholesterol to do so but the mass medication of the will has largely snuffed out the advantage here.

Perhaps we should explore vitamin D in a little more detail and look at other conditions which may appear unrelated to tinnitus but do share an underlying deficiency of vitamin D. Knowing these sometimes helps you make a decision on the causes of your tinnitus and how to address it.

Vitamin D is so vital for health that receptors for this occur in every part of the body. It enhances immune system function produces a broad spectrum antimicrobial called cathelicidin, is anti-inflammatory in nature and strengthens bones by helping the absorption of calcium. That is only a small part of its wonderful ability to keep us healthy.

Vitamin D comes in two forms. One is the inactive form – derived from plant sources (mainly irradiated mushrooms). It is known as vitamin D2 or ergocalciferol.

The active form is known as vitamin D3 or cholecalciferol and is found in but a few food sources. However, most of our vitamin D3 is synthesised from the sun's rays action on the skin.

Poor summers and working indoors, covering up clothing wise or slapping on sun tan lotion all impede our ability to synthesise vitamin D.

Those with dark skins do not synthesise vitamin D well from the sun. The melanin in their skin has a protective effect. From the country of their origin this is necessary in order that the skin does not get damaged. However, if those with darker skins   migrate to a country where the sun is not so intense or shining brightly daily all a year round, then a vitamin D deficiency is likely to occur.

Vitamin D is a fat soluble vitamin. It requires a little fat for absorption so low fat diets hamper absorption into the gut.

These points need to be born in mind because without adequate vitamin D it does not matter how much calcium we take in, it will simply not be absorbed. Even worse, the calcium has to go somewhere but as it cannot gain entry into bones, without vitamin D, then it often gets deposited into joints or in artery linings. Here it starts setting up the initial onset of damaging plaque which is associated with cardiovascular disease.

Elderly people do not absorb nutrients from food as well as they did when they were younger. Stomach acid which aids digestion is much reduced so that food remains partially undigested. Elderly are also inclined to eat less so it is not surprising that osteopenia and osteoporosis are conditions which are generally found in the elderly.

The elderly are often prescribed calcium/vitamin D supplements. These are often chalky white tablets which do nothing for absorption either for vitamin D – which needs to be taken with a little fat – or calcium which requires the help of vitamin D in order to be absorbed.

What is the point of prescribing them? I have to shrug my shoulders at this point. If the prescribing medic does not inform you that they should be taken with a meal that contains some fat, then the prescription is of very little use, if any.

Most people will obtain most of their vitamin D from the sunlight. I will look at this in more detail later.

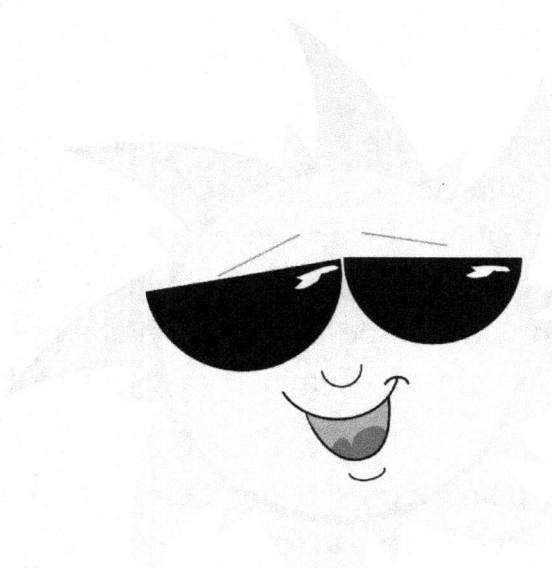

The sun's rays are needed to manufacture vitamin D just under the surface of the skin.

Table showing how serum levels of vitamin D are categorised. (in ng/ml).

Level of vitamin D	Category description
Less than 30 ng/ml	deficient
30-39ng/ml	adequate
40-59ng/ml	optimal
60-100ng/nl	therapeutic
Over 100ng/ml*	

*There aren't actually any consensus standards for vitamin D levels.

Studies in mice who lack vitamin D receptors (known as VDR null mice) show that the main function of vitamin D is to increase calcium absorption from the intestine. However, it also helps the absorption of phosphorus which is also a major player in bone synthesis. I shall return to the role of phosphorus later.

Vitamin D is required to form the hormone calcitriol. Calcitriol is also known as the 'active vitamin D.'

If lack of calcium absorption occurs, then calcium will simply be withdrawn from the bones for any other job it is required for in the body.

Apart from osteopenia and osteoporosis, there are a number of other conditions that point to a vitamin D deficiency. If they occur, then you must consider whether you do have a vitamin D deficiency, ask your GP to test for it or buy your own test from the pharmacy.

These include: bone pain, muscle weakness, fatigue, respiratory infections, diabetes, autoimmune diseases, high blood pressure and mood changes. This is by no means an exhaustive list.

The main foods containing the active form of vitamin D are limited and it is highly unlikely that anyone could take in the recommended daily intake, through diet alone.

Foods containing vitamin D3 (animal origin)

This active form of vitamin D is known as cholecalciferol.

Canned oily fish with the soft bones which should not be discarded as the bones contain calcium. The flesh is the source of vitamin D.

Cod liver oil

Egg yolks

Liver

There is a little vitamin D3 in full fat milk and cheese

Plant sources of vitamin D

The plant based source of vitamin D is known as ergocalciferol.

There are very few sources of vitamin D from plant sources. Really, there is only one contender and that is irradiated mushrooms (mushrooms which have been left out in the sun for half an hour or so). They may contain some vitamin D – in its inactive form - but it is only a very small part of our daily requirement. Therefore, plant eaters use foods – such as fortified plant based milks – in order to increase their intake.

Sunlight as a source of vitamin D

Sunlight, of course – if we can get it – is the best source of vitamin D but it requires adequate amounts of cholesterol which forms part of the structure of skin cells.

Once contact is made by ultra violet B rays with the cholesterol then energy is produced for the synthesis of vitamin D.

This is why vitamin D is known as the 'sunshine vitamin.'

Some people are known to be 'non-responders' to vitamin D. They may pay particular attention to including sufficient vitamin D in their diet but still find they are grossly deficient.

In this scenario, the addition of boron – preferably in the form of calcium fructoborate – appears to overcome this.

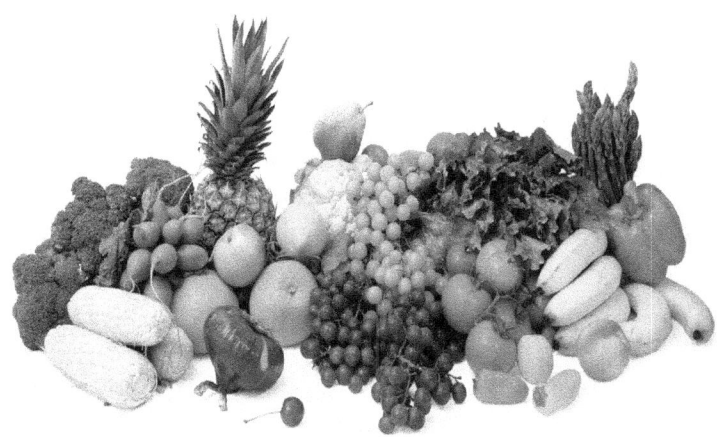

Fruit and veg are great sources of boron which is useful when individuals are non-responders to vitamin D

Storage of vitamin D in the body

Vitamin D is stored in its inactive form in fat cells. When it is required there are two conversion steps needed.

The first step occurs in the liver where the storage form of the liver is converted to calcidiol 1,25(OH)D.

From there it is converted to calcitriol 1,25 (OH) 2D. This occurs mostly in the kidney. This form of vitamin D is the active steroid form.

The active form is the one that attaches itself to Vitamin D Receptors throughout the body. Here it can turn genes on or off.

The genome is more or less permanent. However, there is an epigenome which produces proteins and other molecules which regulate the genes by turning them on or off on the strands of DNA. They are influenced by environmental factors the greatest of these is arguably nutrition and sufficient of the active form of vitamin D.

In the 1950's the incidence of rickets (soft bones which deform easily) was rife. The adult form of rickets is known as osteomalacia and is due to a lack of vitamin D.

To correct this, cod liver oil was recommended. Every school child of that time will recall being given a spoon full of cod liver oil daily.

I did not mind this although most people who lived through these times shudder when recalling it.

A recommended daily intake for vitamin D was issued which was the lowest amount to be taken that could prevent rickets. This was established to be 400 IU's.

While this may be true, it was not widely given out that other systems in the body required much greater amounts to function correctly. For example, the immune system requires about 4000IU's to prevent infection including seasonal virus.

The daily recommended intake would be far too low for elderly adults, who do not absorb nutrients as well, even if they were only considering their bone health and not their overall health.

Such a limited amount of vitamin D would not be of much help to those already grossly deficient and who need to top up quickly.

It would not be of much help to people with malabsorption, dark skin, those staying indoors most of the time, those whose cultures require them to cover their skin up or indeed many other groups who are vulnerable to poor absorption or deficiency of vitamin D for whatever reason.

Calcium does not work in isolation from many other nutrients required for strong, dense bones. A varied diet is essential which includes lots of healthy fats.

Now, the concept of healthy fats may well come unstuck here. Healthy fats are not the vegetable oils that appear to have exploded onto the market. Vegetable oils are not healthy. They are polyunsaturated fatty acids which cause inflammation in the body.

The saturated fats are those from an animal source mainly (although coconut is solid at room temperature and is a saturated fat) and because all the chemical bonds are full, this type of fat is unreactive and cannot cause inflammatory processes.

Furthermore, unlike the plant oils, lard and dripping contain good amounts of vitamin D which the plant oils do not.

Of course, a plant oil that is a monounsaturated fatty acid − a clear exception to the rule − is olive oil. While it does not increase inflammation, it still does not contain vitamin D and we are so very deficient of this in our diets.

The recommended amount of vitamin D3 is 4000I IU's daily, from September to April when the sun rays are not strong.

Provided you are out in the sun from May to August you should obtain enough vitamin D. However, a good rule is that if it is particularly gloomy then take a D3 supplement with a little fat for absorption.

Bear in mind that those who are taking statins, will also have lower cholesterol levels.

Cholesterol is required for the synthesis of vitamin D from the sun's rays.

Cholesterol is also required for the synthesis of bile which helps emulsify fats for better absorption of the fat soluble vitamins. Without this process, fat soluble vitamin D is poorly absorbed. It is difficult enough to get it in your diet anyway, never mind without this added obstacle.

Fluoride inhibits phosphatase in experimental animals and, this enzyme is vital for the absorption of calcium and other minerals. As we have just learned, calcium deficiency was implicated in otosclerosis along with vitamin D.

Supplementing with sodium fluoride found that it halted or slowed the progression of this disease in more than half the patients.

The practice of adding fluoride to domestic water is particularly problematical in many ways. The government excuse that it helps prevent tooth decay is of lesser concern than the myriad of diverse and chronic illness that may occur as a result of mineral deficiencies caused by the addition of fluoride in drinking water and toothpaste. It is hard to find a non-fluoride toothpaste nowadays. Strangely, these appear to be the toothpastes marketed for children's use – the very group that the government are trying to prevent having tooth decay. This doesn't make sense.

In a convoluted way, the addition of fluoride could well be one cause of tinnitus and hearing impairment.

There are tiny amounts of fluoride in tea but the amounts are so small as to be negligible.

Fluoride appears to pay such an important part in hearing impairment that a closer look at this halogen will help aid understanding.

Fluoride is considered to be an essential trace mineral in humans. It was first detected in animals by a gentleman known as Guy Lussac in 1805. Fluorine is the fluoride that is found in trace amounts in bones, the thyroid gland and teeth. It is also found in animal skins as well as human tissue.

Fluorides tend to stay in the extracellular fluid – that is the fluid that surrounds the cells and between 50 and 60% will find its way into bone including the bones in the inner ear. Excess is excreted in the urine. Some fluoride is necessary   for teeth but excessive fluoride is harmful.

Fluoride used therapeutically in sodium fluoride has been used to treat osteoporosis, bone pain (although much bone pain is due to a vitamin D deficiency).

Excessive intakes of fluoride cause a condition called fluorosis. In humans, when the water supply contains more than 10mg fluoride per litre of water, or 110 ppm, an increased density of bone will arise. This is referred to as a sclerosis and it not only affects bone but also supple ligaments in the back which become calcified. Consequently, the condition 'poker back' is manifested. However, it is not just ligaments that are affected but calcification of tendons and muscles also occurs. Thus if you have these symptoms which do not appear related to hearing impairment or tinnitus, then this is a red alert and further investigation should be taken. Now, this is unlikely to be carried out by your GP. This is a responsibility that you must take upon yourself considering all the information that you have. Water boards do not like to be reminded that the addition of fluoride to their water may be detrimental.

China tea also contains huge amounts of fluoride. Each cup of tea will provide 0.5mg of fluoride. Therefore, there could be a connection between tea drinking and otosclerosis and tinnitus. Any increase of bone density due to fluorosis is going to impact nerve transmission in some way which may be interpreted in the multiplicity of sounds found in tinnitus as well as the imposition of a hearing impairment.

Therefore, some steps you could take to ascertain whether you are likely to be suffering from an excessive intake of fluoride is to write to the water board under a Freedom of Information request asking for the amount of fluoride that is put into the water. Remember, it should be no more than

10mg fluoride per litre of water, or 110 ppm,

Then, filter your water. There are filters which work very well and will take your water from your current reading to zero. Our reading used to be 324 ppm so we promptly bought a filter and now it registers zero.

Check for mottled spots on teeth which is a sign of fluorosis.

If you keep having problems with tendons and ligaments or poker back, then this is a further sign of excess intake of fluoride.

Drink less tea.

The **recommended dietary intake of fluoride is just 1mg in the UK as recommended by the Dental Health Committee.**

The ideal drinking water supply is said to be 1mg per litre and while considered to be a reasonable amount for growing children who do not drink tea, it is not so beneficial for adults who do.

Just 4 cups of tea will provide more than double the RDI of fluoride and this does not take into account the fluoride in the water. I am only referring to the fluoride in the tea leaves.

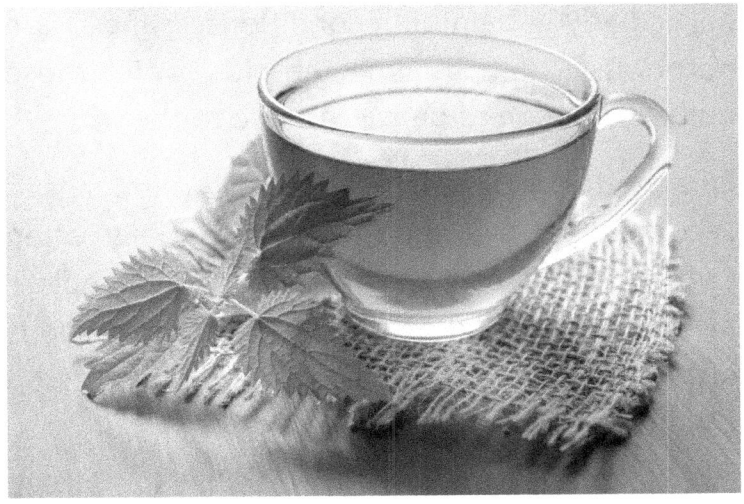

Tea leaves contain excessive amounts of fluoride.

We should now continue with our investigation into the dietary needs of those suffering from hearing impairment and tinnitus. It is well recognised that ear and sinus infection are also related to the above and needs some exploration.

Ear and sinus infection

Ear and sinus infections are often related to some of the vitamin deficiencies that we have already looked at. Sinus and ear infections are particularly painful conditions and are notoriously difficult to get rid of in those unlucky enough to be susceptible to them.

Earache in children is particularly common and accompanied by a deep ache especially when swallowing. It can accompany many sleepless nights for the child as well as the parent who is often up most of the night with a distressed child.

The sinus cavities are a series of hollows in the skull which alleviate the weight of the skull. They do get infected quite easily and often bleed when the infection is severe.

Anyone who has experienced a sinus headache will know how severe they can be. It is impossible to lie down and sleep. Sleep, what you can get of it, must be taken sitting up as any movement forward brings the pain on.

I speak from experience until I discovered vitamin D as a therapeutic agent.

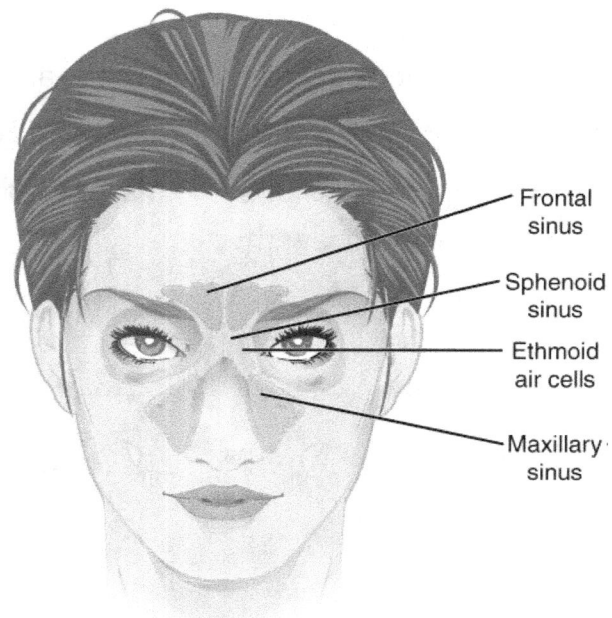

Frontal sinus

Sphenoid sinus

Ethmoid air cells

Maxillary sinus

Vitamin A is needed for healthy mucosal tissue and vitamin D produces an antimicrobial peptide – AMP – which is called cathelicidin and has broad spectrum antimicrobial properties.

Vitamin D is also an activator of the innate immune system – the general defence system that we are born with – as well as activating the acquired immune system which we develop as we come into contact with new infective agents throughout life.

When sinus infection begins, then the immediate therapeutic dosage of 20,000 IU's of vitamin D must be taken with 300mg of magnesium as the activator and some fat for absorption. Do this for at least 3 days or up to a week for stubborn cases of sinusitis.

Zinc supplementation is also useful as zinc is intimately connected with producing enzymes and macromolecules, many of which are required for the smooth running of the immune system.

However, clinical observation of elderly patients with progressive hearing deterioration found that 20% of them had hearing deterioration. These patients did gain some improvement with zinc supplementation. Those with tinnitus noted a reduction – and sometimes an elimination of – tinnitus following supplementation. The improvement did not happen overnight. Damage to serum levels of zinc takes time to address. Supplementation was with zinc sulphate at 600mg daily. After 3 months, serum supplementation was checked and if it fell within normal range of 0.66-1.10 mcg/ml a maintenance dose replaced the above therapeutic dose.

Zinc, of course, is a fairly vulnerable trace mineral. We store only 24 hours' worth of zinc at a time so it is easily depleted with diuretic use. It is another casualty of the ubiquitous proton pump inhibitors being peed out along with so many other vital trace minerals and vitamins. No wonder the elderly suffer so much hearing impairment when they are fed PPI's and diuretics with the enthusiasm they are prescribed.

Electrolyte balances are also known to affect the inner ear. The endolymph has higher levels of potassium and the perilymph higher in sodium. Research has shown that a 24-hour electrolyte urinary clearance test showed that those with sensorineural hearing loss and hypoglycaemia were found to have low sodium levels. After salt had been added to their diet, the sodium potassium balance was restored and hearing improved.

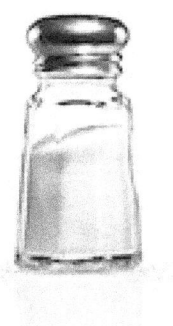

A pinch of salt may improve hearing loss and tinnitus

How is there likely to be an excess of potassium in our diets nowadays? We have largely swung from a carnivorous diet to the recommended 5 or 10 a day. Plant based diets have boomed. Meat is frowned upon. Many of our fruit and vegetables contain high amounts of potassium. Instead of a couple of pieces of fruit a day and maybe a couple of vegetables to go alongside meat, we make smoothies which contain many times the amount of potassium we would normally ingest.   We need sodium to balance potassium.

Of course, we also live in a strange age where we are informed that if we eat too much salt then we will have high blood pressure. A very small percentage of people are salt sensitive and it may affect their blood pressure but there are many more causes of high blood pressure that are absolutely nothing to do with salt. Low salt diets can be just as detrimental to health as high salt diets. Moderation is the key.

A small amount of sodium is needed to conduct nerve impulses – those very impulses that eventually end up in the auditory cortex to be interpreted into something we find intelligible. If is needed to maintain a proper balance of water and minerals. Many people report tinnitus when prescribed diuretics because diuretics rid the body of many essential minerals including sodium.

Post chemo. Its constant! Sounds like i am stuck between channels on an old FM radio. Then there's the intermittent high pitch squealing in either ear. Need constant white noise to drown it out. No such thing a quiet anymore

Louise

Both potassium and sodium work together to make sure that the fluid balance in the body is exactly right. As we age, this may be more difficult to balance although many other nutrients which are found in excess or deficient may contribute to an imbalance in fluid balance.

Diuretics are well known for causing hearing loss. They induce pathological change in the cochlear. Furosemide induces temporary hearing loss unless other risk factors are present which compound any hearing impairment or tinnitus. Some of the impact is due to the action of the diuretic which, when it reduces fluid volume, also causes vasoconstriction. We have already looked at vasoconstriction in relation to the action of adrenalin in those suffering from stress. It is a risk factor for tinnitus.

The cochlea is fairly well protected from toxic matter but when local vasoconstriction occurs, an ischaemia is prompted and the protection is lost. This is only transient but the entry of toxic matter or bacteria, for example, will disrupt the clean vibratory flow of nerve impulses which would cause fluctuating hearing impairment and tinnitus.

As you can see there is a whole host of reasons why tinnitus and hearing impairment occur and each require a bespoke response. Dehydration would also induce some hearing loss due to vasoconstriction caused by loss of fluid. Here are some more below.

In 2001 just after I'd had my ears syringed. Initially just in my right ear but eventually in both. Noise like a 56k modem. Hearing aids have helped enormously TBF.

Lee Holme

My tinnitus is low level and I only hear it when all is quiet. It's high-pitched and slightly a different tone in each ear. Started after platinum-based chemotherapy in 2016.

Daveymidds

I have severe ME. & my tinnitus is constant, high pitched. I can deal with this ok but when I'm in a crash/relapse it is worse & a loud screeching sound. I'm noise sensitive due to M.E. & it's a noise I can't switch off when I need to the most

Sunnydays 4071

I have suffered tinnitus for 15 years. I also have exploding head syndrome. It is a sleep disorder related to tinnitus. It scared the life out of me initially until I understood what it was.

Suzanne

I suffered for about 6 months following a head injury, I found it unbearable. I don't know how people cope and dread it ever coming back. Mine was like a really loud pulsating noise, drove me bonkers. My heart goes out to any one suffering. Makes me really appreciate silence

Katy

It doesn't attract any sympathy. The standard response is " it's nothing to do with AZ". Funny it only became almost unbearable after my first jab of AZ, which has now been withdrawn? The eyes are more of a problem for me and the tinnitus is more bearable since having aids fitted

Ian Huggins

I had my hair washed in a salon 23 years ago and leaning my head against the backwash really hurt and my ears rang. It has never stopped.

Call Me Hennimore

I experienced tinnitus for a short time when I had severe anaemia. A few transfusions later I was ok.

Michele John

My dad has it but it's music he hears ….. he describes it as Russian opera….. always in the background

Mrs T

I woke up in the surgery recovery room hearing a buzzing sound following orbital decompression surgery in 2008. It's still buzzing.

Cubicle 17

Mine was like whooshing noises inside my head, going through phases like cycles of a washing machine. I think mine was due to B12 deficiency (B12 tabs only work if you absorb it). Much better since I started self-injecting, but other symptoms are taking forever to improve.

AEMoerbeek

The symptoms of dehydration are fairly easy to spot so it is useful to memorise them as it may be useful when investigating hearing impairment and tinnitus for yourself or others. We will temporarily turn our attention to this subject

Dehydration

Dehydration occurs when more fluid is lost than what is taken in. You need sufficient fluids in order for body systems to work properly and without it serious complications can occur.

Mild dehydration results in headache and irritability and generally a feeling of thirst although the thirst reflex may be lost in the elderly. Dehydration may also occur because due to age and infirmity, they cannot actually physically access water.

Hot and humid weather increases the risk of dehydration. The process of sweating causes evaporation to occur and this takes some of the heat from the body.

Elderly people tend to have fewer fluid reserves in their body. Chronic illness such as dementia and diabetes, some medications, like diuretics, can all disrupt the fluid balance. Gastrointestinal upset which involve diarrhoea or vomiting will also disturb the fluid balance and can impact auditory status.

Individuals involved in sport who do not rehydrate regularly or replace their electrolytes may find that they suffer hearing impairment and tinnitus   Electrolytes really are very important because once the normal cell to cell signalling is disrupted then odd though it may seem, it can impact hearing as well as any other system in the body.

Symptoms of dehydration can include:

Low blood pressure

Increased heart rate (tachycardia)

Dry mouth and tongue

Deeply sunken eyes and cheeks

Irritability and general lassitude

Dark coloured urine

Dizziness and/or confusion

Headache

If you take the skin at the back of your hand and pinch it gently, it should snap back fairly rapidly in those who are not dehydrated.

Contributors to dehydration include:

Vomiting and diarrhoea

Heat stroke and excessive sun

Alcohol

Excessive exercising

A fever

Diuretic use

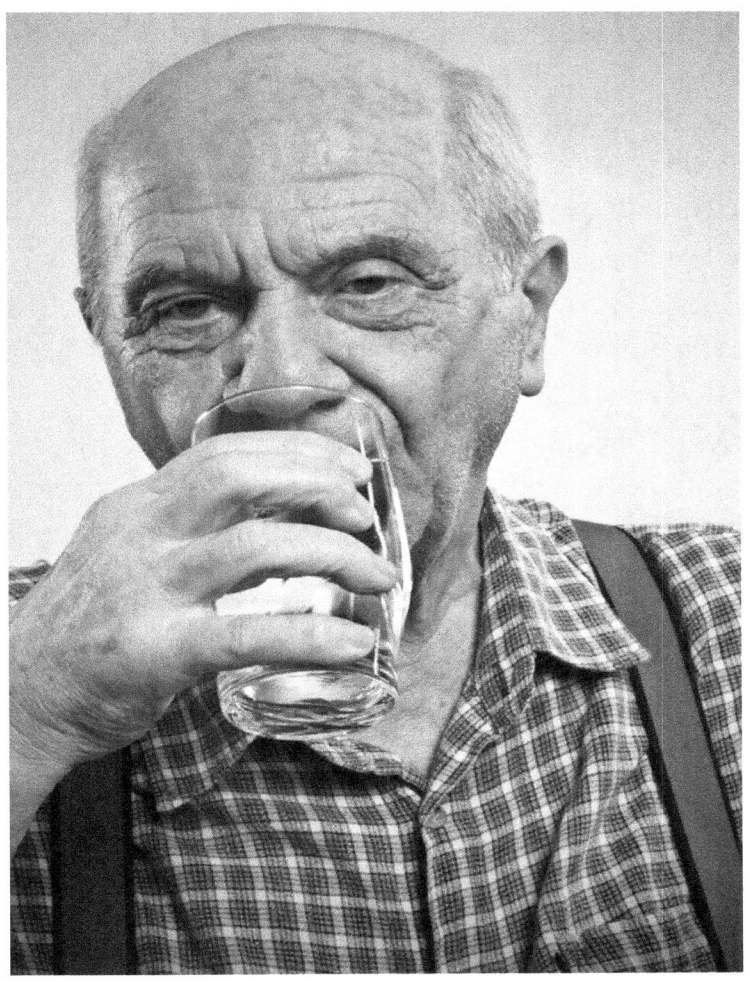

The elderly should get into the habit of taking in about 1 litre of fluid a day. Excessive amounts will just leach vital nutrients from their body. Food also contains water and they will be taking in more than you think.

Another source of [7]secondary tinnitus – the tinnitus which is caused by a specific underlying cause - may be due to a vitamin B12 deficiency which is a very common condition generally confined to the elderly.

There may be a number of reasons for this which may include:

Weak stomach acid. Vitamin B12 needs an acidic environment in order for it to be separated from its protein source. The elderly generally has insufficient acid and it tends not to be as acidic as it would be when younger. This may be because there is a deficiency of vitamin B1 which is required to release acid from gastric cells.

Poor dental care may mean that many foods which contain vitamin B12 are not eaten. Red meat is an excellent source of this vitamin but chewing may be a problem. In this case, beef

---

[7] Primary tinnitus is referred to as idiopathic in that it has no known cause whilst secondary tinnitus will have an identifiable underlying cause.

may be taken minced which would allow for a greater surface area and subsequent absorption.

A lack of motivation to make meals or eat the end result.

Vitamin B12 and folate deficiency

In 1933, researchers Shemesh et al found that tinnitus patients often had a vitamin B12 deficiency. Supplementation was found to help.

A good vascular supply is need for optimum cochlear function and for the proper functioning of nervous tissue. When a vitamin B12 deficiency exists there is demyelination of the nerves, axonal degeneration and eventually programmed cell death.

The myelin sheath around nerves is needed to transmit impulses and any disruption to this action in the nerves that serve the cochlear and auditory centre will have the potential to disrupt normal hearing. Thus demyelination in the cochlear area will also negatively impact hearing.

Folate and vitamin B12 deficiency are linked to the destruction of the tiny blood vessels found in the stria vascularis and the distortion or loss of hearing.

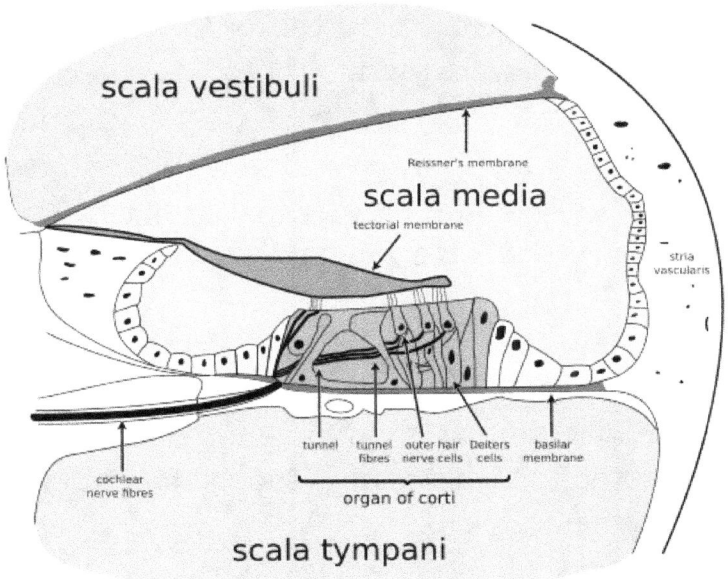

scala vestibuli

Reissner's membrane

scala media

tectorial membrane

stria
vascularis

cochlear
nerve fibres

tunnel   tunnel   outer hair   Deiters   basilar
          fibres   nerve cells   cells   membrane

organ of corti

scala tympani

In order to evidence the impact of a deficiency of vitamin B12 on hearing, a study was carried out to look at the prevalence of tinnitus in an Indian population who reported chronic, subjective tinnitus.

To avoid the problems of absorption, vitamin B12 injections were used.

The pilot study was carried out at Lucknow Medical College for one year from August 2012. The patients were aged between 18-60 years old.

Chronic tinnitus was defined as being present for more than 6 months and clearly was considered to be distressing enough for patients to seek medical help.

Both genders were included and the main exclusion was those with pulsatile tinnitus or those with congenital abnormalities which might account for tinnitus symptoms.

Other exclusions included:

Those with psychiatric illness

Anyone suffering an ear infection

Those with acoustic injury or had been exposed to chronic noise

Those suffering from systemic disease such as diabetes, thyroid dysfunction, hypertension, anaemia.

Anyone who had been on medication known to impact hearing, for the past four weeks. These would include vasodilators and steroids.

Anyone who had tinnitus after a head injury

Twenty patients were allocated to Group A and another twenty allocated to Group B. Group A receiver parenteral intramuscular vitamin B12 of 2500mcg weekly for 6 weeks. Group B were given a placebo of saline intramuscularly for the same length of time.

The observations were analysed. Self- reported questionnaires were also used.

The results showed that those in Group A who had a pre-existing deficiency of vitamin B12 showed significant improvement after 6 weeks of intramuscular vitamin B12. Those who did not have a deficiency of B12 did not show improvement.

In Group B, no improvement was noted in any patient.

Therefore, the study showed that vitamin B12 deficiency, once corrected improved the subjective experience of those with tinnitus.

My Tinnitus came following 3 weeks of Covid 19. NOT a vaccine injury- as I declined the jabs. As i was recovering I got 1/2 a day of vertigo, it went & was replaced my bi-lateral tinnitus. High pitched sounds sometimes wake me up at night. I am seeing a medical herbalist.

John

It's awful hearing ringing, swishing and different notes whistling in my head. Nothing I've done seems to help. Tried all the "exercises and videos" out there to make it better. Along with vertigo this sucks the most...

Aunt Molly

I've had it for years & it's getting worse. I feel like I can hear my own nervous system & sometimes I hear feelings. It's definitely electrical. I have various noises at different pitches in both ears & it affects my hearing.

Suzy Boots

I get varying tones that also feel more musical. Mine are not constant, though.

Ethereum Suzy

I have constant noises going up and down in volume. Both ears. Usually high pitched like tuning in a radio in the old days. It affects my hearing when it is loud.

Carole Rogers

Dementia, deafness, dietary deficiency and tinnitus

It has been recognised that there is a link between deafness and dementia. It has been recognised for decades that a deficiency of B vitamins – in particular niacin (vitamin B3) is a major risk factor for dementia.

Robust research shows that tinnitus and some hearing impairment precedes Parkinson's disease and Alzheimer's disease.

Early onset dementia is found among those with tinnitus.

In 2021 YF Chang carried out a study on 2616 patients with pre-existing tinnitus. He found that pre-existing tinnitus was associated with a whopping 68% increased risk dementia after he had adjusted for socio demographic characteristics and medical comorbidities.

It may be that the tinnitus ran concurrently with some subtle subclinical changes that occur in early onset dementia but it often preceded neurodegenerative disorders like Parkinson's disease and Alzheimer's.

Although niacin deficiency is a risk factor for dementia, the other B vitamins have equal importance. Vitamin B1 – thiamine – impacts the whole of the body being a vital cofactor in the mitochondria.

Mitochondria are the powerhouse in every cell in the body. They convert glucose (from our food) and oxygen into energy revving up each cell's ability to function at optimum speed. However, thiamine is the spark plug that actions this. Without thiamine nothing can be initiated and unfortunately, thiamine is a hidden deficiency in society.

We do know that amyloid beta protein is found in the brains of those with Alzheimer's disease and equally we know that once a thiamine deficiency is corrected the plaques begin to dissolve and are removed. If dementia is caught at the early stages and treated with thiamine, then cognitive function may return. What has this to do with tinnitus?

Some studies[8] have shown that administering thiamine intravenously may alleviate deafness which was caused by such a deficiency. Thiamine appears to stabilise the nervous system as a whole but with greater specificity in the inner ear.

Thiamine does work rapidly and as it has no upper tolerable limit, can be taken in large doses. Those with Parkinson's disease are often prescribed 3g daily. The recommended dosage is 1.4mg daily but I believe this is far too low in today's climate. However, dosage as high as 3g are not required in tinnitus where there does not appear to be overt dementia. Doses of 100mg-500mg will suffice.

Thiamine needs to be activated and its activator is magnesium. Without magnesium it will be

---

[8] https://www.ncbi.nlm.nih.gov/pmc/articles/PMC3970335/

useless. Any B vitamin used in higher therapeutic doses needs to be accompanied by a good vitamin B complex as well.

Niacin is needed for the proper breakdown of the macromolecules, protein, fat and carbohydrate. Another of its functions is to aid the smooth working of the central nervous system.

Pellagra is the condition caused by a deficiency of niacin. Pellagra's later stages are manifested in a form of dementia. However, there is only limited research showing that niacin deficiency is associated with tinnitus. The link between pellagric dementia and tinnitus in this case is not clear. It is quite likely that if the central nervous system is impacted by niacin deficiency then this is likely to include the auditory cortex but studies are sparse on this subject and not hugely significant.

Niacin can damage kidneys if taken in large doses so therapeutic doses are not recommended. The niacin included in a B complex supplement should be enough.

Pyroxidone is vitamin B6. Like all B vitamins it is water soluble and, as such, needs to be taken in diet on a daily basis as it is not stored in the body.

The B vitamins are very much characterised by their ability to produce energy from the breakdown of fats, protein and carbohydrate and pyroxidone is no different. In addition, it helps in the synthesis of hormones, some enzymes and red blood cells. It is needed in the production of the feel good neurotransmitter, serotonin. It helps sleep, reduces sensitivity to pain, acts as an important cofactor in many biological pathways. It is ant sickness and can be used as a travel sickness remedy or morning sickness. It is known as the ant depressive vitamin and it has a good reputation for addressing tinnitus.

Most B vitamins are found in similar foods. Thus beef liver, salmon, tuna, fortified cereals, poultry, chickpeas, dark green leafy vegetables, like spinach, wholemeal foods, wheat germ and similar are all good sources of the B vitamins.

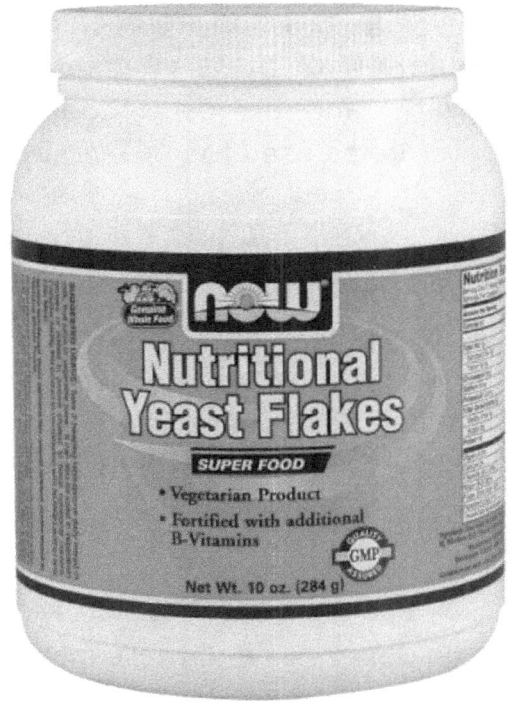

Nutritional yeast flakes are an excellent source of the B vitamins

Thiamine is more likely to be found in pork muscle meats and pork liver than beef but the other sources apply to the whole of the complex.

B vitamins tend to degrade rapidly with sunlight, cooking, heat and storage. As they are water soluble any of these vitamins will leach into the water and be lost. Cooking water should therefore be used to make gravy.

If one B vitamin is known to be deficient then it is highly likely that the others are too. This is a nutritional complex that I do recommend is supplemented on a daily basis once individuals are over the age of 50 years. The B vitamins are a remarkable complex which address so many of the allegedly 'age related' conditions.

There are some conditions that increase the risk of vitamin B6 deficiency and these include:

Autoimmune intestinal conditions like Crohn's disease and ulcerative colitis

Autoimmune inflammatory disorders like rheumatoid arthritis

Alcoholism

Kidney disease

There is also anecdotal evidence that folate (synthetic form is folic acid) can help stabilise the nervous system.

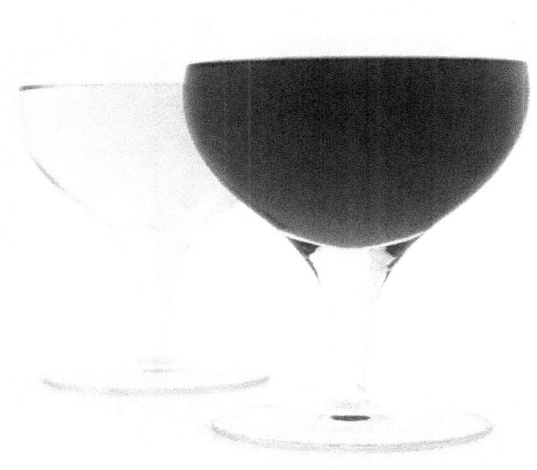

Too much alcohol can not only deplete vitamin B6 but is known to degrade thiamine rapidly. Both of these vitamins are vital for optimum cochlear status

there are much more interesting studies that show that high homocysteine levels are a risk factor for premature hearing loss. It is folic acid that prevents the build-up of homocysteine and by preventing the mechanisms which can cause oxidative stress.

Homocysteine is an amino acid which is required – briefly – to participate in the methionine cycle. It is broken down in the presence of vitamins B6, folate and vitamin B12. Without these in sufficient quantities homocysteine can cause a build-up of plaque in the arteries.

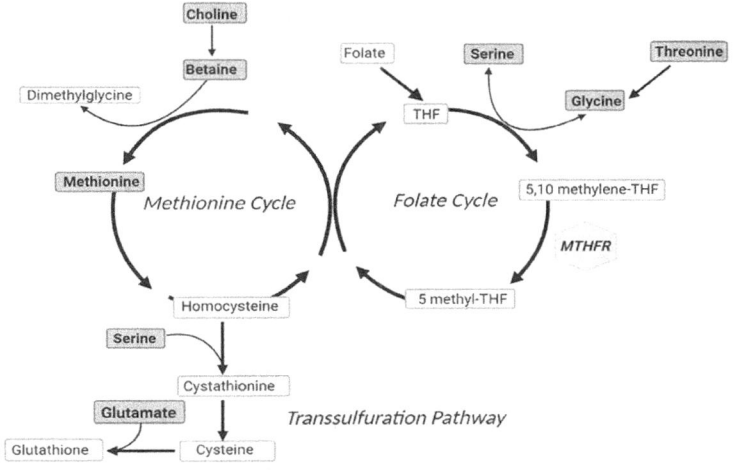

The methionine cycle requires homocysteine only briefly to complete its cycle. Homocysteine is broken down with B6, folate and vitamin B12

When arteries are disrupted through vasoconstriction such as that would occur due to plaque lining the microvasculature, the electrical activity arriving at the auditory cortex will determine the volume and pitch of the tinnitus experienced.

It is clear that the elevated homocysteine that is associated with dementia, stroke and heart disease has the potential to be comorbid with hearing impairment and tinnitus due to the high homocysteine levels than can underpin them both.

The exact cause of tinnitus and related hearing impairment is still a puzzle for many. We know that the neural activity is disrupted but there is no clear consensus why.

However, looking for one cause detracts from the fact that tinnitus is not a condition but a symptom which can have many an underlying cause.

We have learned from the many voices that have appeared in this book that tinnitus is characterised by a range of noises some of which may be permanent and other pulsating or temporary. Each of these manifestations can give us a clue as to what is causing a person's tinnitus.

The fact that it appears to be prevalent in older people suggests a degenerative process which often occurs due to a nutritional deficiency whether due to poor nutrition or poor absorption. Both of these are correctable with a little thought. Sometimes, a month's supplementation of the B vitamins can provide enough energy to motivate someone to want to cook for themselves again.

The description of tinnitus can be somewhat clumsy and heavy going.

The neurophysiological model of lastreboff described it as

A subcortical perception and results from the processing of weak neural activity in the periphery. The tinnitus related neural activity occurring usually near the periphery of the system undergoes processing in subcortical auditory pathways and finally perceived at a conscious level as sound.

It is stated that there is no treatment for tinnitus primarily because the underlying cause is not clear. However, I would argue that the underlying causes are generally clear and often related to nutritional deficiency.

Where tinnitus is related to trauma or infection, chemo or some other non-innate cause, there is always the potential for improvement and recovery. It is a gross insult to patients to inform them that they will probably have to live with a condition, which is distressing, for the rest of their lives. The impact on sleep and concentration, when it is lifelong, decrease the quality of life severely.

It is however, the progression of what is deemed an innocuous symptom, into an overt neurodegenerative disorder, that is most troubling. This can be stopped if caught early and the cause addressed but for some reason it is not.

There are treatments which tend to mask the symptoms or help patients cope with the tinnitus but this is not good enough. Masking does not prevent the progression into a neurodegenerative disorder, neither does learning coping strategies when counselling is offered.

What are the popular treatments on offer?

Hearing aids - generally used for patients with hearing loss and tinnitus

Counselling – it is mooted that understanding what causes the hearing loss and tinnitus makes it more bearable. Statements from many do not bear this out.

Table top sound generators play nature sounds like falling rain or waterfalls. This has been said to help people fall asleep.

 Most doctors will offer a combination of the treatments below, depending on the severity of your tinnitus and the areas of your life it affects the most.

Wearable sound generators fit into the ear and use similar sounds to that found in the table top generators to detract from the tinnitus.

For those whose tinnitus is very loud acoustic neural stimulation may be used. This consists of a small device which stimulates the neural circuits and allegedly desensitises the patient to the tinnitus. This appears to have had some success in eliminating tinnitus. My question is though, has it eliminated the underlying damage that caused the tinnitus in the first place. How did it achieve that? If the original damage has not been undone, then is there not a danger that subclinical damage is still occurring and is not being addressed in its early stages?

Antidepressants may be prescribed but do nothing for the disorder underpinning the tinnitus and hearing impairment. The correct response would be to correct the reason for the tinnitus. Antidepressants do not come without their own problems and are a risk factor for dementia too as has recently been raised in the media. The 'hungover' effect that they produce also reduces the quality of life.

Cochlear implants bypass the damaged part of the inner ear. Direct electrical signals are sent to stimulate the auditory nerve. Cochlear implants are generally used in those patients who have severe hearing loss. However, it tells us little about what the original cause of the hearing loss was or how we could correct it.

Although nutritional deficiencies have been explored and are found to correct or improve tinnitus or hearing impairment, this research is not recent and has been overshadowed by invasive methods such as hyperactivity and deep brain stimulation.

It seems to me that we have become a nation of guinea- pigs. Some of the new treatments are not necessary but they do gain a lot of research funding. The humble nutrient – whether vitamin, mineral or macromolecule is not seen as the answer when more often than not, it is the only effective answer.

We still have not learned that ageing is a process of changes but it does not include pain or degeneration which is often considered to go hand in hand with a

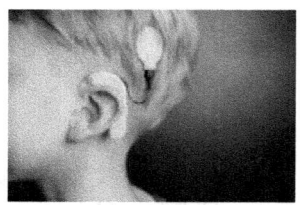

A cochlear transplant in a young boy

advancing age. How long will it take for people to understand that this is not the case? How long will people accept this erroneous assumption and allow themselves to be subjected to all manner of atrocities when simple nutritional changes are sometimes all that is needed?

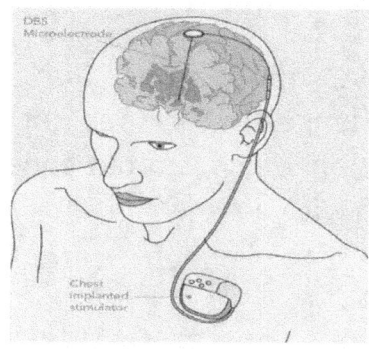

Deep brain stimulation is sometimes used for hearing impairment.

Finally, the most common cause of tinnitus and hearing impairment is the build-up of ear wax.

The build-up of ear wax does not appear particularly problematical in the young. The wax in the young is soft and yellowish. In older people, especially in those who have damaged ear canals where some narrowing has occurred with the addition of hair inside them (another phenomenon which appears in later life) then the wax appears darker and less soft.

Other contributors to ear wax build-up is a scalp infection or inner ear infection often referred to as 'swimmer's ear.

The contributory cause must be addressed alongside the softening and removal of the ear wax. Nothing should be inserted inside the ear canal as it is more likely to push the wax further in and cause further problems.

A few drops of warmed olive oil inserted into the ear twice daily until the wax softens and dislodges itself will benefit this process. Olive oil is anti-inflammatory in nature and will address any inflammatory processes going on inside.

The whole process should be gentle and carried out for the minimum amount of time. Once the wax is removed, hearing is restored instantly. The procedure may need to be repeated at annual intervals or sooner if the individual is finding it hard to hear at any point.

We have now come to the end of the book on tinnitus, hearing impairment and dietary influences on the above.

It is an important subject because the impairment or tinnitus is indicative of much more serious subclinical pathologies. If you can find the cause of the tinnitus and address it then it is quite likely that pathological changes occurring elsewhere are also being addressed.

I am minded that in Parkinson's disease, that by the time symptoms are manifested – such as tremor – that 80% of the brain associated with

Parkinson's disease has already been affected. Tinnitus has the potential to be a much earlier warning sign which, if investigated with the time and attention that it deserves, may prevent a full blown manifestation of more serious disease.

Finally, when any condition of nervous origin manifests itself, although healing will begin straight away if the correct nutrients are ingested, nerves may take a longer time to heal than other tissues.

Every tissue has its own healing time. The gut lining may take less than 24 hours to replace damaged cells. Skin takes approximately a week; nerves can take up to a year. This may explain why people think that nerves cannot repair themselves. They can, it just takes a little longer.

Some dementias will respond to the Thiamine Regime

300mg of thiamine

300mg of magnesium

A good vitamin B complex

Plus, add in 3g of L-taurine daily

Superfoods

Liver – beef, pigs and lamb (lightly cooked)

Organ meats in general

Yeast flakes, yeast extract, brewer's yeast

Eggs

Bone broths

Full fat dairy milk and butter

Protocol for sinus and ear infection

At the first sign of infection take

20,000 IU's of vitamin D

300mg of magnesium

50mg of zinc

3g of vitamin C in divided doses

continue this for up to one week

Other books by this author include:

- The EDS and Hypermobility Syndrome Diet
- Alleviating Symptoms of EDS
- Gastroparesis
- The EDS recipe book
- The Lipoedema Diet
- The Lymphoedema Diet: reverse and repair lymphatic damage
- The Anti-Virus Diet
- The Asthma Diet
- The Reluctant Bowel
- The MND Diet
- Why we live longer with higher cholesterol levels
- A dietary connection for MACS, POTS and EDS

- Identity: a self-exploration workbook *
- Journey Through Pneumonia
- Parkinson's Disease: dietary changes that work
- The Thyroid Diet
- https://www.amazon.co.uk/dp/B07TBHM V6N

*This book can be used alone or in small group work and is an excellent resource for those who are 'people helpers.'

Among many others

They are available on Amazon

Lynne has written a semi-autobiographical trilogy.

For the full range of books by this author, visit the author website on

https://www.amazon.co.uk/-/e/B07BPQZ5CD

https://www.amazon.com/-/e/B07BPQZ5CD

A percentage of the profits from the sale of these books go to support charities like the Exodus Project below.

The Exodus Project

My first introduction to the far reaching impact of The Exodus Project occurred when I was travelling around Cawthorne in one of their buses, visiting gardens. A young lad was happily munching on a sandwich. He looked up briefly, pointed to the driver and said,' He's my second dad, he is,' then he returned to his sandwich without further comment

Such remarks are often very telling and so I arranged to meet Jackie Peel and Martin Sawdon, at the charity's premises in Barnsley. They set up the Exodus Project 20 years ago. They moved into their current premises — a redundant Methodist church - in 2010.

Both Jackie and Martin have been youth workers in their church. Martin worked in housing for the homeless in addition to working in learning disabilities services in institutional settings.

The work that the Exodus Project undertakes is of paramount importance to the communities it serves. These were former mining communities which became disadvantaged after pit-closures. Currently about 400 children attend mid-week activities from Monday to Thursday inclusive. These activities include dance, drama, craft, music, sports and games. In addition, there are weekend camps, cycle treks, outward bound activities, bowling and swimming. The children are taught valuable life skills including how to cook and bake. It is all about teaching children how to fulfil their potential and learn skills they will be able to pass onto the next generation.

The grounds, once overgrown, have been turned into a play- and camping - ground. A miniature railway is in the process of being installed.

Martin and Jackie have developed a unique model in that The Exodus Project goes beyond dispensing services. They are keen to build up relationships with the whole family and not just the child that attends the mid- week clubs. In addition, once children have reached the age of fourteen, they are invited to help out with the younger groups as junior volunteers. Once they reach the age of eighteen, they become adult volunteers. This model provides a constant supply of help from individuals who have benefitted already from attending such groups.

The building is large and inviting. It is decorated with bold colours and has comfy seating. It is a real home from home; a haven for families who have been disadvantaged by the closure of the life force of its community.

Martin and Jackie have clear ideas about how they wish to develop the Exodus Project but the lottery funding which they benefitted from is no longer available. Sadly, they have had to close two of their clubs due to lack of funding. This decision wasn't taken lightly. They do have two charity shops which raises some money and they obtain some funding from outside organisations for the use of their facilities. However, this is clearly not enough to keep their clubs, weekend activities and building going to cater for the ever growing number of children who are benefitting from the work being undertaken here.   Neither does it allow for future development.

Exodus do have a Just Giving page which can be found here if you wish to help further their work https://www.justgiving.com/exodus

In addition, you can keep up with activities on their Facebook page here

https://www.facebook.com/search/top/?q=the%20exodus%20project%20barnsley&epa=SEARCH_BOX

Recommended small businesses

https://skinkiss.org.uk/

https://favouritekafei.co.uk/?fbclid=IwAR1pW2
OJNWCtFdIpgU7WWp9JQiQDxbBxu4GfzBfr6648
snFYFERRYvGW7Ss

www.ingramcontent.com/pod-product-compliance
Lightning Source LLC
Chambersburg PA
CBHW070559220526
45467CB00003B/1252